Consume
To
Overcome your Diet

A comprehensive Guide to Healthy Eating
and Sustainable Weight loss

By
Frankly L Williams

Introduction

In a world inundated with fad diets, quick-fix solutions, and conflicting nutritional advice, the quest for sustainable weight management and optimal health can often feel like an uphill battle. "Eat to Beat Your Diet" offers a refreshing approach to achieving your wellness goals by empowering you with the knowledge and tools to make informed dietary choices that nourish your body, fuel your vitality, and support long-term well-being.

Table of Content

- Delving into the fundamentals of metabolism, energy balance, and body composition
- Exploring the role of macronutrients (carbohydrates, proteins, and fats) in supporting overall health and satiety
- Highlighting evidence-based strategies for achieving and maintaining a healthy weight

Chapter 3: Nourishing Your Body with Whole Foods

- Celebrating the abundance and diversity of nutrient-rich whole foods
- Providing practical tips for incorporating more fruits, vegetables, whole grains, lean proteins, and healthy fats into your diet

- Emphasizing the importance of mindful eating and savoring the sensory experience of food

Chapter 4: Building Balanced Meals and Snacks

- Offering guidance on portion control, meal planning, and mindful eating habits
- Providing sample meal plans and recipe ideas for creating balanced, satisfying meals
- Exploring the concept of intuitive eating and listening to your body's hunger and fullness cues

Chapter 5: Making Informed Food Choices in a Busy World

- Navigating the grocery store aisles with confidence and discernment
- Decoding food labels and marketing claims to make informed purchasing decisions
- Offering practical strategies for dining out, traveling, and managing social situations while staying true to your health goals

Chapter 6: Cultivating Sustainable Lifestyle Habits

- Recognizing the interconnectedness of nutrition, physical activity, sleep, stress management, and overall well-being
- Providing evidence-based recommendations for incorporating movement, relaxation techniques, and

self-care practices into your daily routine
- Empowering you to make sustainable lifestyle changes that support your health and vitality for the long haul

Chapter 7: Overcoming Challenges and Staying Motivated

- Identifying common obstacles to healthy eating and weight management
- Offering practical solutions for overcoming setbacks, managing cravings, and staying motivated on your journey
- Fostering a supportive community and mindset of self-compassion, resilience, and perseveran.

CHAPTER 1
UNDERSTANDING THE PITFALL OF DIET

Exploring the limitations and drawbacks of traditional dieting approach

Exploring the limitations and drawbacks of traditional dieting approaches is essential for why many people struggle to achieve long-term success with weight management and overall health. Traditional dieting typically involves restrictive eating patterns, calorie counting, and short-term goals focused solely on weight loss. While these approaches may yield initial results, they often fail to address the root causes of unhealthy eating habits and can lead to a variety of negative consequences. Let's delve into some of the key limitations and drawbacks of traditional dieting:

Unsustainability:

1. Traditional diets often rely on extreme restrictions or elimination of certain food groups, making them difficult to maintain over the long term. This can lead to feelings of deprivation, cravings, and ultimately, rebound weight gain once the diet is discontinued.

Focus on External Factors:

2. Traditional diets tend to prioritize external factors such as calorie

counts, portion sizes, and rigid meal plans, rather than addressing internal cues such as hunger, fullness, and emotional eating. This disconnect from internal signals can contribute to a disordered relationship with food and a lack of mindfulness around eating habits.

Nutrient Deficiencies:

3. Many traditional diets promote overly restrictive eating patterns that may result in nutrient deficiencies, particularly if certain food groups are eliminated. This can lead to fatigue, weakened immunity, and other health complications over time.

Negative Psychological Effects:

4.   The restrictive nature of traditional diets can have negative psychological effects, including increased stress, anxiety, and feelings of guilt or shame associated with food choices. This can perpetuate a cycle of emotional eating and unhealthy coping mechanisms.

Yo-Yo Dieting:

5.   Traditional dieting often leads to a pattern of yo-yo dieting, where individuals cycle between periods of strict adherence to a diet and subsequent lapses into overeating or binge eating. This cycle of weight loss and regain can have detrimental

effects on metabolism, body composition, and overall health.

Lack of Individualization:

6. Traditional diets tend to offer one-size-fits-all approaches that may not take into account individual differences in metabolism, lifestyle, cultural preferences, and medical conditions. This lack of personalization can hinder long-term adherence and success.

Focus on Appearance Over Health:

7. Many traditional diets prioritize achieving a certain aesthetic appearance (such as thinness or muscularity) over promoting overall health and well-being. This emphasis on external appearance can

perpetuate harmful body image ideals and undermine self-esteem.

In summary, exploring the limitations and drawbacks of traditional dieting approaches highlights the need for a shift towards more holistic, sustainable, and individualized approaches to health and nutrition. By focusing on nourishing the body with nutrient-rich foods, cultivating mindful eating habits, and addressing the underlying factors driving unhealthy behaviors, individuals can achieve lasting success in achieving their health and wellness goals.

 driving unhealthy behaviors, individuals can achieve lasting success in achieving their health and wellness goals.

Unveiling the Myth and Misconceptions Surrounding Weight Loss and Diet.

Unveiling the myths and misconceptions surrounding weight loss and diet culture is crucial for promoting a more informed and balanced approach to health and wellness. Diet culture, which perpetuates unrealistic ideals of thinness, promotes restrictive eating patterns, and prioritizes external appearance over overall well-being, is rife with myths and misconceptions that can harm individuals physically, mentally, and emotionally. Let's explore some of these myths and misconceptions in detail:

1.   **Myth: Rapid Weight Loss Equals Success:**
   - One of the most pervasive myths perpetuated by diet culture is that rapid weight loss is the key indicator of success. However, rapid weight loss is often unsustainable and can lead to muscle loss, nutrient deficiencies, and metabolic slowdown, ultimately resulting in rebound weight gain in the long term.
2.   Myth: All Calories Are Created Equal:
   - Another common misconception is that weight loss is simply a matter of calories in versus calories out. While energy

balance is important, not all calories are created equal in terms of their impact on metabolism, hunger, and overall health. The quality of the foods consumed, including their nutrient density and macronutrient composition, plays a significant role in weight management and overall well-being.

3. **Myth: Carbohydrates Are the Enemy:**
   - Carbohydrates have long been vilified by some diet plans as the culprit behind weight gain and metabolic disorders. However, not all carbohydrates are created equal, and whole food sources of

carbohydrates, such as fruits, vegetables, and whole grains, are essential for providing energy, fiber, vitamins, and minerals. It's refined carbohydrates and excessive sugar intake that are more closely linked to adverse health outcomes.

4. **Myth: Fat-Free Equals Healthy:**
   o The fat-free craze of the 1990s perpetuated the myth that eliminating fat from the diet was the key to weight loss and optimal health. However, not all fats are harmful, and certain types of fats, such as monounsaturated and polyunsaturated fats found in nuts, seeds, avocados, and fatty

fish, are essential for supporting brain function, hormone production, and cardiovascular health.

5. **Myth: Exercise Alone Can Counteract Poor Diet:**
    - While exercise is undoubtedly important for overall health and weight management, it cannot compensate for a poor diet. The saying "you can't out-exercise a bad diet" holds true, as nutrition plays a primary role in determining body composition and overall well-being. A balanced approach that combines regular physical activity with a nutrient-rich diet is essential for

achieving optimal health outcomes.

6. **Myth: Health Looks a Certain Way:**
   - Diet culture often promotes a narrow definition of health based solely on external appearance, equating thinness with wellness and moral virtue. This narrow focus overlooks the diversity of body shapes and sizes and ignores the importance of factors such as genetics, socioeconomic status, and access to resources in shaping health outcomes.

Unveiling these myths and misconceptions surrounding weight loss and diet culture is essential for promoting a more nuanced and compassionate understanding of health and wellness. By challenging these harmful beliefs and adopting a more holistic approach that prioritizes nourishment, self-care, and body acceptance, individuals can cultivate a healthier and more sustainable relationship with food, exercise, and their bodies.

Emphasizing the Importance of Adopting a Holistic, Lifestyle-centered Approach to Health and Nutrition

Emphasizing the importance of adoptinga holistic, lifestyle-centered approach to health and nutrition is fundamental for promoting long-term well-being and vitality. Unlike traditional dieting approaches that focus solely on short-term weight loss goals, a holistic approach considers the interconnectedness of various aspects of health, including nutrition, physical activity, sleep, stress management, and emotional well-being. Let's explore the key components and benefits of a lifestyle-centered approach to health and nutrition:

1. **Nutritional Quality:** Rather than solely focusing on calorie counting or restricting certain food groups, a holistic approach prioritizes the quality of the foods consumed. This involves emphasizing whole, minimally processed foods that are nutrient-dense and support overall health. By nourishing the body with a variety of fruits, vegetables, whole grains, lean proteins, and healthy fats, individuals can optimize their intake of essential vitamins, minerals, antioxidants, and phytonutrients.
2. **Mindful Eating:** Mindful eating is a core principle of a lifestyle-centered

approach to nutrition. It involves paying attention to hunger and fullness cues, savoring the sensory experience of eating, and cultivating a nonjudgmental awareness of thoughts, emotions, and behaviors related to food. By practicing mindful eating, individuals can develop a healthier relationship with food, reduce emotional eating, and improve digestion and satisfaction with meals.

3. **Physical Activity:** Regular physical activity is essential for overall health and well-being, and a lifestyle-centered approach emphasizes finding enjoyable forms of exercise that fit into one's daily routine. Whether it's walking, cycling, yoga, strength training, or

recreational sports, incorporating movement into daily life can improve cardiovascular health, muscle strength, flexibility, mood, and energy levels.

4.   **Stress Management:** Chronic stress can have a profound impact on physical and mental health, affecting everything from appetite and digestion to immune function and inflammation. A lifestyle-centered approach to health and nutrition recognizes the importance of stress management techniques such as mindfulness meditation, deep breathing exercises, yoga, and relaxation techniques in promoting resilience, emotional balance, and overall well-being.

5.   **Sleep Hygiene:** Quality sleep is essential for optimal health and functioning, yet it is often overlooked in discussions of nutrition and wellness. A lifestyle-centered approach emphasizes the importance of prioritizing sleep hygiene practices such as maintaining a regular sleep schedule, creating a restful sleep environment, and practicing relaxation techniques before bedtime. Adequate sleep supports cognitive function, mood regulation, immune health, and metabolic balance.

6.   **Social Connection and Support:** Human connection and social support play a vital role in promoting health and well-being. A lifestyle-centered approach recognizes the

importance of fostering meaningful relationships, cultivating social support networks, and engaging in activities that bring joy and fulfillment. Whether it's sharing meals with loved ones, participating in group fitness classes, or volunteering in the community, social connection contributes to overall happiness and resilience.

7.   **Self-Care:** Self-care encompasses a range of activities and practices that nourish the mind, body, and spirit. This may include practicing gratitude, setting boundaries, engaging in hobbies, spending time in nature, and prioritizing activities that promote relaxation and rejuvenation. By prioritizing self-care, individuals can

reduce stress, enhance self-esteem, and cultivate a greater sense of balance and fulfillment in life.

In summary, emphasizing the importance of adopting a holistic, lifestyle-centered approach to health and nutrition recognizes that true wellness encompasses more than just physical health or appearance. By addressing various aspects of health, including nutrition, physical activity, stress management, sleep, social connection, and self-care, individuals can cultivate a balanced and sustainable approach to living that promotes vitality, resilience, and overall well-being.

CHAPTER 2
THE SCIENCE OF SUSTAINABLE WEIGHT MANAGEMENT

Delving into the fundamentals of metabolism, energy balance, and body composition

Delving into the fundamentals of metabolism, energy balance, and body composition is essential for understanding how our bodies process nutrients, regulate energy expenditure, and maintain overall health. These interconnected processes play a critical role in determining body weight, composition, and metabolic health. Let's explore each of these fundamentals in more detail:

1. **Metabolism**:
   - Metabolism refers to the complex biochemical processes that occur within the body to convert food into energy. It encompasses two main components: anabolism, which involves the synthesis of molecules to build and repair tissues, and catabolism, which involves the breakdown of molecules to release energy.
   - Basal metabolic rate (BMR) represents the energy expended by the body at rest to maintain basic physiological functions such

as breathing, circulation, and cell repair. Factors that influence BMR include age, gender, body composition, muscle mass, and genetics.

- **Thermic effect of food (TEF)** refers to the energy expended during digestion, absorption, and metabolism of nutrients. Different macronutrients have varying TEFs, with protein requiring the most energy to digest, followed by carbohydrates and fats.
- **Physical activity level (PAL)** accounts for the energy expended through structured exercise, daily activities, and non-exercise thermogenesis (NEAT), which

includes activities such as walking, fidgeting, and standing.

2. **Energy Balance:**

- Energy balance is the relationship between energy intake (calories consumed from food and beverages) and energy expenditure (calories burned through metabolism and physical activity). It is the primary determinant of changes in body weight and composition.
- When energy intake exceeds energy expenditure, a positive energy balance occurs, leading to weight gain and potentially alterations in body composition (e.g., increased fat mass).

Conversely, when energy expenditure exceeds energy intake, a negative energy balance occurs, resulting in weight loss and potential changes in body composition (e.g., loss of fat mass and/or lean mass).

- Energy balance is influenced by a multitude of factors, including dietary choices, portion sizes, meal frequency, macronutrient composition, physical activity patterns, metabolic rate, hormones, and environmental factors.

3. **Body Composition:**

- Body composition refers to the proportion of fat, muscle, bone, and other tissues that comprise the body. It is a more meaningful indicator of health than body weight alone, as it reflects the distribution of lean mass and fat mass.

- Lean body mass (LBM) includes muscles, bones, organs, and connective tissues, while fat mass (FM) represents adipose tissue stored throughout the body. A healthy body composition is characterized by an appropriate ratio of lean mass to fat mass.
- Body composition can be assessed using various methods, including dual-energy X-ray absorptiometry (DEXA),

bioelectrical impedance analysis (BIA), skinfold calipers, and waist circumference measurements. These techniques provide valuable insights into overall health, metabolic risk, and fitness levels.

- Achieving and maintaining a healthy body composition requires a balanced approach that includes regular physical activity, resistance training to preserve lean muscle mass, adequate protein intake, and a nutrient-dense diet that supports metabolic health.

In summary, delving into the fundamentals of metabolism, energy balance, and body composition provides a comprehensive understanding of how our bodies regulate energy, utilize nutrients, and maintain overall health. By optimizing these processes through mindful eating, regular physical activity, and lifestyle modifications, individuals can achieve sustainable weight management, improve metabolic health, and enhance overall well-being.

Exploring the role of macronutrients (carbohydrates, proteins, and fats) in supporting overall health and satiety.

Exploring the role of macronutrients—carbohydrates, proteins, and fats—in supporting overall health and satiety is essential for understanding how different dietary components contribute to our nutritional needs, energy levels, and feelings of fullness. Each macronutrient serves unique functions in the body and plays a crucial role in supporting various physiological processes. Let's delve into the roles of carbohydrates, proteins, and fats in more detail:

1. **Carbohydrates:**
   - Carbohydrates are the body's primary source of energy, providing approximately 4 calories

per gram. They are found in a wide variety of foods, including grains, fruits, vegetables, legumes, and dairy products.

- Carbohydrates are broken down into glucose, which serves as the main fuel for cells throughout the body, particularly the brain and muscles.

- In addition to providing energy, carbohydrates play a vital role in supporting overall health by supplying fiber, vitamins, minerals, and phytonutrients. Fiber, in particular, is essential for digestive health, regulating blood sugar levels, and promoting feelings of fullness and satiety.

- Choosing complex carbohydrates, such as whole grains, fruits, vegetables, and legumes, over refined carbohydrates (e.g., white bread, sugary snacks) can help stabilize blood sugar levels, reduce cravings, and support long-term energy levels.

2. Proteins:

- Proteins are essential for building and repairing tissues, synthesizing enzymes and hormones, and supporting immune function. They are composed of amino acids, which are often referred to as the building blocks of life.

- Unlike carbohydrates and fats, proteins are not stored in the body for energy but are instead used for structural and functional purposes.
- Including adequate protein in the diet is crucial for supporting muscle health, promoting satiety, and aiding in weight management. Protein-rich foods such as lean meats, poultry, fish, eggs, dairy products, legumes, nuts, and seeds can help regulate appetite, increase metabolism, and preserve lean muscle mass during weight loss.
- Consuming a balanced mix of essential amino acids from

various protein sources is important for supporting optimal health and meeting the body's protein requirements.

3. **Fats:**

- Fats are a concentrated source of energy, providing approximately 9 calories per gram. They play a vital role in supporting cell structure and function, hormone production, nutrient absorption, and insulation.

- Dietary fats are classified into saturated fats, unsaturated fats (including monounsaturated and polyunsaturated fats), and trans fats. Unsaturated fats, particularly omega-3 and omega-6 fatty acids found in fatty fish, nuts, seeds, and plant oils, are considered heart-healthy and essential for brain health.

- Including healthy fats in the diet can enhance feelings of satiety and promote long-lasting energy levels. Fat slows down the digestion process, which helps regulate appetite and prevents spikes in blood sugar levels.
- Choosing sources of healthy fats, such as avocados, olive oil, nuts, seeds, and fatty fish, can help reduce the risk of chronic diseases such as heart disease, diabetes, and obesity.

In summary, exploring the role of macronutrients in supporting overall health and satiety underscores the importance of consuming a balanced diet that includes a variety of nutrient-dense foods. By incorporating carbohydrates, proteins, and fats in appropriate proportions, individuals can optimize energy levels, support metabolic health, and promote feelings of fullness and satisfaction after meals. Additionally, focusing on whole, minimally processed foods and mindful eating practices can further enhance the nutritional quality of the diet and contribute to long-term well-being.

Highlighting evidence-based strategies for achieving and maintaining a healthy weight

Highlighting evidence-based strategies for achieving and maintaining a healthy weight is crucial for individuals seeking sustainable approaches to weight management. These strategies are grounded in scientific research and emphasize lifestyle modifications that promote long-term success rather than quick-fix solutions. Let's explore some evidence-based strategies in detail:

1. **Balanced Diet:**
   - Adopting a balanced diet that emphasizes whole, nutrient-dense foods is essential for achieving and maintaining a healthy weight. Focus on incorporating plenty of fruits, vegetables, whole grains, lean proteins, and healthy fats into your meals and snacks.
   - Aim to consume a variety of foods from different food groups to ensure you're getting a wide range of essential nutrients. This approach helps promote satiety, regulate blood sugar levels, and support overall health.

- Be mindful of portion sizes and practice intuitive eating by listening to your body's hunger and fullness cues. Avoid strict calorie counting or restrictive eating patterns, as these can lead to feelings of deprivation and unsustainable habits.

2. **Regular Physical Activity:**

- Engaging in regular physical activity is crucial for achieving and maintaining a healthy weight. Aim for at least 150 minutes of moderate-intensity aerobic exercise or 75 minutes of vigorous-intensity exercise per week, along with muscle-strengthening activities on two or more days per week.

- Find activities that you enjoy and incorporate them into your daily routine. This could include walking, jogging, cycling, swimming, dancing, or participating in group fitness classes.
- Remember that physical activity is not just about burning calories; it also provides numerous other health benefits, including improved mood, increased energy levels, and reduced risk of chronic diseases.

3. **Mindful Eating:**

- Practicing mindful eating can help you develop a healthier relationship with food and support weight management goals. Pay attention to your body's hunger and fullness cues, eat slowly, and savor the flavors and textures of your food.
- Avoid distractions while eating, such as watching TV or scrolling on your phone, as these can lead to mindless overeating. Instead, focus on the sensory experience of eating and tune in to how different foods make you feel physically and emotionally.
- Be mindful of emotional eating triggers and find alternative

coping mechanisms, such as
practicing relaxation techniques,
journaling, or seeking support
from friends and family.

4. **Behavioral Changes:**
   - Adopting behavior-based
     strategies can help you make
     lasting changes to your eating
     and activity habits. Set realistic,
     achievable goals, and track your
     progress over time. Celebrate
     your successes and learn from
     setbacks without being too hard
     on yourself.
   - Identify potential barriers to
     healthy eating and physical
     activity, such as time constraints,
     stress, or social pressures, and

develop strategies to overcome them. This may involve meal planning, scheduling workouts, enlisting support from friends or family, or seeking guidance from a healthcare professional or registered dietitian.

- Focus on building sustainable habits that align with your values and preferences rather than following strict rules or fad diets. Remember that small, consistent changes over time can lead to significant improvements in weight and overall health.

5. **Support System:**

- Surround yourself with a supportive network of friends,

family, or peers who encourage and motivate you on your weight loss journey. Share your goals with others and seek out accountability partners who can help keep you on track.

- Consider joining a weight loss support group, attending wellness workshops, or working with a registered dietitian or certified health coach who can provide personalized guidance and support.
- Remember that everyone's journey to a healthy weight is unique, and it's essential to find the strategies and approaches that work best for you. Be patient

with yourself, stay committed to your goals, and focus on progress rather than perfection.

In summary, highlighting evidence-based strategies for achieving and maintaining a healthy weight involves adopting a balanced diet, engaging in regular physical activity, practicing mindful eating, making behavior-based changes, and seeking support from others. By incorporating these strategies into your lifestyle and staying committed to long-term habits, you can achieve sustainable weight management and improve your overall health and well-being.

CHAPTER 3
NOURISHING YOUR BODY WITH WHOLE FOOD

Celebrating the Abundance and

Diversity of Nutrient rich Foods

Celebrating the abundance and diversity of nutrient-rich whole foods is a cornerstone of promoting optimal health, vitality, and well-being. Whole foods are those that are minimally processed and retain their natural integrity, providing a rich array of essential nutrients, vitamins, minerals, fiber, antioxidants, and phytonutrients. Embracing a diet rich in whole foods allows individuals to nourish their bodies with the diverse array of nutrients needed for optimal function and vitality. Let's delve into the importance and benefits of celebrating

the abundance and diversity of whole
foods:

1. **Nutrient Density:**
    - Whole foods are inherently
      nutrient-dense, meaning they
      contain a high concentration of
      essential nutrients relative to their
      caloric content. Fruits, vegetables,
      whole grains, legumes, nuts,
      seeds, lean proteins, and fatty fish
      are all examples of nutrient-rich
      whole foods.
    - By incorporating a variety of
      whole foods into your diet, you
      can ensure that you're meeting
      your body's nutritional needs and
      supporting overall health. Each
      food offers a unique profile of

vitamins, minerals, and phytonutrients that contribute to various aspects of health and well-being.

2. **Diverse Array of Nutrients:**
    - Whole foods come in a diverse array of colors, flavors, and textures, each indicative of the unique nutrients they contain. For example, brightly colored fruits and vegetables are rich in antioxidants such as vitamin C, beta-carotene, and anthocyanins, which help protect against oxidative stress and inflammation.
    - Including a rainbow of fruits and vegetables in your diet ensures that you're getting a wide range of

nutrients that support immune function, heart health, brain health, and more. Aim to eat a variety of colors each day to maximize your intake of essential nutrients and phytochemicals.

3. **Fiber-Rich Foods:**
   - Many whole foods are excellent sources of dietary fiber, which is important for digestive health, blood sugar regulation, cholesterol management, and weight management. Fiber-rich foods such as fruits, vegetables, whole grains, legumes, nuts, and seeds help promote feelings of fullness and satiety, which can aid in weight control.

○ Including plenty of fiber-rich foods in your diet supports a healthy gut microbiome, enhances regularity, and reduces the risk of chronic diseases such as heart disease, diabetes, and certain cancers.

4. **Minimally Processed:**
   ○ Whole foods are minimally processed and retain their natural integrity, unlike processed and ultra-processed foods, which often contain added sugars, unhealthy fats, artificial additives, and preservatives. By choosing whole foods over processed options, you can minimize your intake of added sugars, sodium, and

unhealthy fats while maximizing your intake of essential nutrients.

- Opting for whole foods in their natural state allows you to enjoy the pure flavors and nutritional benefits of fresh, wholesome ingredients. Whether it's a crisp apple, a vibrant salad, or a nourishing bowl of homemade soup, whole foods offer a sensory experience that processed foods cannot replicate.

5. **Environmental Sustainability:**
   - Embracing a diet rich in whole foods supports environmental sustainability by reducing reliance on heavily processed, resource-intensive foods and promoting the

consumption of locally grown, seasonal produce. Whole foods tend to have a lower environmental footprint compared to processed foods, which often require extensive processing, packaging, and transportation.
  - Choosing locally sourced, organic, and sustainably produced whole foods whenever possible helps protect natural ecosystems, conserve resources, and support local farmers and producers.

6. **Culinary Creativity:**
   - Celebrating the abundance and diversity of whole foods opens up a world of culinary possibilities and encourages creativity in the

kitchen. Experimenting with different ingredients, flavors, and cooking techniques allows you to discover new tastes and textures while nourishing your body with wholesome, flavorful meals.

- Whether you're exploring global cuisines, trying out new recipes, or incorporating seasonal produce into your meals, embracing whole foods can inspire a lifelong journey of culinary exploration and enjoyment.

In summary, celebrating the abundance and diversity of nutrient-rich whole foods is essential for promoting optimal health, vitality, and well-being. By embracing whole foods as the foundation of your diet, you can nourish your body with the diverse array of nutrients needed for optimal function, support digestive health and regularity, reduce the risk of chronic diseases, and cultivate a deeper connection to the natural world and the food you eat. Let whole foods be your inspiration and guide on the path to vibrant health and culinary delight.

Providing Pratical Tips For Incorporating More Fruits, Vegetables

Whole grains, Lean protein and Healthy Fats in Your Diet

Incorporating more fruits, vegetables, whole grains, lean proteins, and healthy fats into your diet is essential for promoting overall health, supporting weight management, and reducing the risk of chronic diseases. These nutrient-rich foods provide essential vitamins, minerals, antioxidants, fiber, and phytonutrients that support optimal function of the body. Here are some practical tips for incorporating these foods into your diet:

1. **Fruits and Vegetables:**
   - Aim to include a variety of fruits and vegetables in your meals and snacks throughout the day. Choose a rainbow of colors to ensure you're getting a wide range of vitamins, minerals, and phytonutrients.
   - Keep a bowl of fresh fruit on your kitchen counter or desk for easy snacking. Apples, bananas, oranges, berries, and grapes are convenient options that require minimal preparation.
   - Add vegetables to omelets, stir-fries, soups, salads, and pasta dishes to boost flavor, texture, and nutritional value. Experiment

with different cooking methods, such as roasting, steaming, grilling, or sautéing, to enhance the taste and appeal of vegetables.

- Incorporate vegetables into smoothies and juices for a nutrient-packed beverage. Leafy greens, such as spinach and kale, blend well with fruits and provide an extra boost of vitamins and minerals.
- Keep frozen fruits and vegetables on hand for quick and convenient meal preparation. Frozen produce is just as nutritious as fresh and can be easily added to smoothies, stir-fries, soups, and casseroles.

2. **Whole Grains:**

- Choose whole grains such as brown rice, quinoa, barley, oats, bulgur, farro, and whole wheat bread, pasta, and tortillas over refined grains. Whole grains are higher in fiber, vitamins, and minerals and provide sustained energy throughout the day.
- Start your day with a nutritious breakfast featuring whole grains. Enjoy oatmeal topped with fresh fruit and nuts, whole grain toast with avocado or nut butter, or whole grain cereal with milk or yogurt.
- Swap out refined grains for whole grains in your favorite recipes.

Use whole wheat flour in baking, substitute brown rice for white rice, or try whole grain pasta in pasta dishes.

- Experiment with ancient grains such as quinoa, farro, and amaranth in salads, grain bowls, and side dishes. These nutrient-rich grains add variety and texture to your meals while providing essential nutrients.

3. **Lean Proteins:**

- Include a source of lean protein in each meal and snack to support muscle health, promote satiety, and regulate blood sugar levels. Lean protein options include poultry, fish, seafood, lean cuts of beef or pork, tofu, tempeh, legumes, eggs, and low-fat dairy products.

- Plan meals around protein-rich foods, such as grilled chicken breast, baked fish, lentil soup, or tofu stir-fry. Add protein to salads by topping them with grilled shrimp, hard-boiled eggs, or chickpeas.
- Incorporate plant-based proteins into your diet by trying meatless meals a few times a week. Experiment with vegetarian dishes such as bean chili, lentil curry, black bean tacos, or quinoa salads.

- Use portion control when serving protein-rich foods to avoid overeating. Aim for a palm-sized portion of protein at each meal, and balance it with plenty of vegetables and whole grains for a well-rounded meal.

4. **Healthy Fats:**

- Choose sources of healthy fats such as avocados, nuts, seeds, olive oil, coconut oil, fatty fish (salmon, mackerel, sardines), and nut butters. These fats provide essential fatty acids, vitamins, and antioxidants that support heart health and brain function.
- Incorporate avocado into sandwiches, salads, wraps, and

smoothies for a creamy texture and rich flavor. Spread avocado on whole grain toast and top with sliced tomatoes and a sprinkle of sea salt for a simple and satisfying snack.

- Snack on a handful of nuts or seeds for a quick and nutritious pick-me-up. Almonds, walnuts, pistachios, chia seeds, and flaxseeds are excellent sources of healthy fats, protein, and fiber.
- Use olive oil or avocado oil for cooking and salad dressings to add flavor and healthy fats to your meals. Drizzle olive oil over roasted vegetables or use it to sauté greens for a tasty side dish.

- Include fatty fish in your diet at least twice a week to boost your intake of omega-3 fatty acids. Grill or bake salmon, mackerel, or sardines and serve them with a side of roasted vegetables and quinoa for a nutritious meal.

In summary, incorporating more fruits, vegetables, whole grains, lean proteins, and healthy fats into your diet is essential for supporting overall health and well-being. By including a variety of nutrient-rich foods in your meals and snacks, you can provide your body with the essential nutrients it needs to thrive. Experiment with different ingredients, flavors, and cooking techniques to make healthy eating enjoyable and sustainable for the long term. Remember that small changes can lead to big results over time, so start by making one or two changes at a time and gradually build on your progress.

Emphasing the Importance of Mindful And Savouring the Sensory Experience of Food

Emphasizing the importance of mindful eating and savoring the sensory experience of food is a key aspect of fostering a healthier relationship with food, promoting overall well-being, and cultivating a greater appreciation for the nourishment that food provides. Mindful eating involves bringing awareness and attention to the present moment while consuming food, allowing for a deeper connection with the sensory aspects of eating. Let's explore the significance of mindful eating and practical ways to incorporate it into daily life:

1. **Enhanced Awareness:**
    - Mindful eating encourages heightened awareness of physical hunger and fullness cues, as well as emotional and environmental triggers for eating. By tuning into these cues, individuals can make more conscious choices about when, what, and how much to eat, rather than relying on external cues or unconscious eating habits.

- Practicing mindfulness during meals and snacks allows individuals to savor the flavors, textures, and aromas of food, enhancing the eating experience and promoting greater satisfaction and enjoyment.

2. **Reduced Overeating:**

- Mindful eating can help prevent overeating and promote more balanced eating habits by encouraging individuals to eat in response to hunger and fullness signals rather than external factors such as portion sizes, social pressures, or emotional triggers.

- By slowing down and paying attention to the physical sensations of hunger and satiety, individuals are better able to recognize when they are truly hungry and when they have had enough to eat, leading to more mindful and intuitive eating patterns.

3. **Improved Digestion:**

- Eating mindfully can support better digestion and nutrient absorption by allowing the body to fully engage in the digestive process. Chewing food thoroughly, savoring each bite, and eating in a relaxed environment promotes optimal digestion and reduces the risk of digestive discomfort such as bloating or indigestion.

- Mindful eating also encourages individuals to pay attention to how different foods make them feel physically and emotionally, helping them make more informed choices about food selection and portion sizes to support digestive health.

4. **Emotional Well-Being:**

- Mindful eating can have positive effects on emotional well-being by promoting greater self-awareness, self-compassion, and resilience in the face of stress or emotional eating triggers. By cultivating a nonjudgmental attitude toward food and eating habits, individuals can develop a healthier relationship with food and reduce feelings of guilt, shame, or anxiety surrounding eating.

- Engaging in mindful eating practices, such as deep breathing, mindful chewing, and body scans, can help individuals manage stress, regulate emotions, and cultivate a greater sense of calm and balance in their lives.

5. **Cultivation of Gratitude:**

- Savoring the sensory experience of food can foster a greater sense of gratitude for the abundance and variety of flavors, textures, and colors that nature provides. Taking the time to appreciate the journey of food from farm to table, as well as the effort and care that goes into its cultivation and preparation, can deepen one's connection to food and foster a sense of gratitude for the nourishment it provides.

- Practicing gratitude during meals and snacks can enhance the eating experience and promote a more positive relationship with food and body image.

6. **Practical Tips for Mindful Eating:**

- Eat slowly and chew food thoroughly, paying attention to the taste, texture, and aroma of each bite.
- Minimize distractions while eating, such as television, smartphones, or reading material, to fully engage in the eating experience.
- Pause before and during meals to check in with your hunger and fullness cues, as well as your emotional state.
- Take deep breaths and practice relaxation techniques before meals to promote a sense of calm and presence.
- Use all your senses to fully experience the food—notice the

colors, smells, sounds, and textures of each dish.
- Express gratitude for the food you are about to eat and the nourishment it provides to your body and mind.

In summary, emphasizing the importance of mindful eating and savoring the sensory experience of food can lead to a deeper appreciation of the nourishment that food provides, promote healthier eating habits, and enhance overall well-being. By cultivating mindfulness during meals and snacks, individuals can develop a greater awareness of their eating patterns, reduce overeating, support digestion, manage emotions, and foster a more positive relationship with food and body image. Mindful eating is not about perfection but rather about cultivating presence, curiosity, and kindness toward oneself and the eating experience.

CHAPTER 4
BUILDING BALANCED MEALS AND SNACKS

Offering guidance on portion control, meal planning, and mindful eating habits

Offering guidance on portion control, meal planning, and mindful eating habits is essential for promoting balanced and sustainable eating patterns, supporting overall health, and achieving nutrition goals. These practices empower individuals to make informed choices about their food intake, manage portion sizes effectively, and develop a healthier relationship with food. Let's explore each of these components in detail:

1. **Portion Control:**
   - Portion control involves managing the amount of food consumed in a single sitting to meet nutritional needs without overeating. It's important to recognize that portion sizes can vary depending on individual factors such as age, gender, activity level, and metabolic rate.
   - Use visual cues and portion size guidelines to estimate appropriate serving sizes. For example, a serving of protein (such as meat, poultry, or fish) is roughly the size

of your palm, a serving of grains
(such as rice or pasta) is about
the size of your fist, and a serving
of vegetables is about the size of
your clenched fist.

- Practice mindful eating by paying
  attention to hunger and fullness
  cues to determine when to start
  and stop eating. Eat slowly,
  savoring each bite, and pause
  occasionally to check in with your
  body's signals of hunger and
  satiety.

- Be mindful of portion distortion,
  which occurs when oversized
  portions become the norm and
  can lead to overeating. Avoid
  super-sized or jumbo portions at

restaurants and opt for smaller-
sized options when available.

2. **Meal Planning:**

   - Meal planning involves preparing
     meals and snacks ahead of time
     to support healthy eating habits
     and streamline the cooking
     process. It can help save time,
     money, and stress while
     promoting balanced nutrition and
     portion control.

   - Set aside time each week to plan
     your meals and snacks, taking
     into account your schedule,
     nutritional needs, and
     preferences. Consider
     incorporating a variety of foods

from all food groups to ensure a balanced diet.

- Create a grocery list based on your meal plan and stick to it while shopping to avoid impulse purchases of unhealthy foods. Choose fresh, whole ingredients whenever possible and limit processed and convenience foods.
- Batch cook and pre-portion meals and snacks for the week to make healthy eating more convenient and accessible. Divide larger dishes into individual portions and store them in reusable containers for easy grab-and-go options.

3. **Mindful Eating Habits:**

- Mindful eating involves bringing awareness and attention to the present moment while eating, allowing for a deeper connection with the sensory experience of food. It encourages individuals to eat with intention, attention, and curiosity.
- Start each meal with a moment of gratitude or reflection to cultivate a positive mindset and set the tone for mindful eating. Take a few deep breaths to center yourself and bring your focus to the present moment.
- Notice the colors, textures, aromas, and flavors of your food as you eat, engaging all your

senses in the eating experience. Chew slowly and thoroughly, savoring each bite, and pay attention to how the food makes you feel physically and emotionally.
  ○ Practice nonjudgmental awareness of thoughts, feelings, and sensations related to eating, without labeling them as good or bad. Be compassionate toward yourself and your body, recognizing that eating is a natural and necessary part of life.

By offering guidance on portion control, meal planning, and mindful eating habits, individuals can develop healthier eating patterns, achieve their nutrition goals, and cultivate a more balanced and sustainable relationship with food. These practices empower individuals to make informed choices about their food intake, manage portion sizes effectively, and develop a healthier relationship with food. By incorporating these strategies into their daily routine, individuals can support overall health and well-being and enjoy the benefits of mindful and nourishing eating habits.

Providing Sample Meal Plans and Recipe Ideas for Creating Balanced, Satisfying Meals

Providing sample meal plans and recipe ideas for creating balanced, satisfying meals is a valuable tool for individuals looking to improve their nutrition, manage their weight, and cultivate healthier eating habits. These meal plans offer practical guidance on incorporating a variety of nutrient-rich foods into daily meals and snacks while promoting portion control and mindful eating practices. Let's explore some sample meal plans and recipe ideas for creating balanced, satisfying meals across different dietary preferences and lifestyles:

Sample Meal Plan 1: Mediterranean-Inspired Meal Plan

Day 1:

- Breakfast: Greek yogurt parfait with mixed berries, honey, and granola
- Lunch: Mediterranean quinoa salad with cucumber, tomatoes, feta cheese, olives, and a lemon-herb vinaigrette
- Dinner: Grilled lemon herb chicken served with roasted vegetables (bell peppers, zucchini, eggplant) and whole grain couscous
- Snack: Hummus with sliced bell peppers and whole grain crackers

Day 2:

- Breakfast: Spinach and feta omelet with whole grain toast
- Lunch: Falafel wrap with hummus, tabbouleh, cucumber, and tzatziki sauce, served with a side of Greek salad
- Dinner: Baked salmon with roasted potatoes and green beans, drizzled with olive oil and herbs
- Snack: Greek yogurt with sliced peaches and a sprinkle of cinnamon

Sample Meal Plan 2: Plant-Based Meal Plan

Day 1:

- Breakfast: Overnight oats made with almond milk, chia seeds, and mixed berries

- Lunch: Quinoa and black bean salad with avocado, corn, tomatoes, cilantro, and lime dressing
- Dinner: Vegan chickpea curry with spinach, served over brown rice
- Snack: Sliced apples with almond butter

Day 2:

- Breakfast: Smoothie bowl topped with banana slices, shredded coconut, and hemp seeds
- Lunch: Lentil and vegetable soup with whole grain bread
- Dinner: Stir-fried tofu with mixed vegetables (bell peppers, broccoli, carrots) and teriyaki sauce, served over quinoa
- Snack: Carrot sticks with hummus

Sample Meal Plan 3: High-Protein Meal Plan

Day 1:

- Breakfast: Scrambled eggs with spinach, tomatoes, and feta cheese, served with whole grain toast
- Lunch: Grilled chicken Caesar salad with romaine lettuce, cherry tomatoes, Parmesan cheese, and Caesar dressing
- Dinner: Baked tilapia with quinoa pilaf and roasted asparagus
- Snack: Greek yogurt with sliced almonds and honey

Day 2:

- Breakfast: Protein smoothie made with whey protein powder, banana, spinach, and almond milk

- Lunch: Turkey and avocado wrap with lettuce, tomato, and mustard, served with a side of carrot sticks
- Dinner: Beef stir-fry with broccoli, bell peppers, and snap peas, served over brown rice
- Snack: Cottage cheese with pineapple chunks

Recipe Ideas:

- Grilled Vegetable Quinoa Bowl: Grilled vegetables (such as zucchini, bell peppers, eggplant) served over cooked quinoa, drizzled with balsamic glaze and topped with fresh herbs and crumbled feta cheese.
- Sweet Potato and Black Bean Tacos: Roasted sweet potato slices and black beans stuffed into whole grain

tortillas, topped with avocado slices, salsa, and cilantro.

- Mango Avocado Salad: Mixed greens topped with diced mango, avocado slices, red onion, and toasted pumpkin seeds, dressed with a lime vinaigrette.
- Salmon and Asparagus Foil Packets: Salmon fillets and asparagus spears seasoned with lemon, garlic, and herbs, wrapped in foil and baked until tender.
- Quinoa-Stuffed Bell Peppers: Bell peppers filled with cooked quinoa, black beans, corn, diced tomatoes, and spices, topped with shredded cheese and baked until bubbly.

Incorporating these sample meal plans and recipe ideas into your weekly rotation can help you create balanced, satisfying meals that support your nutritional needs and taste preferences. Experiment with different ingredients, flavors, and cooking techniques to keep meals exciting and enjoyable while nourishing your body with wholesome, flavorful foods. Remember to practice portion control, mindful eating, and moderation to maintain a healthy and balanced diet.

Exploring the Concept of Intuitive Eating and Listening to Your Body's Hunger and Fullness Cues

Exploring the concept of intuitive eating and listening to your body's hunger and fullness cues is a transformative approach to eating that emphasizes self-awareness, mindfulness, and trust in one's internal signals of hunger, fullness, and satisfaction. Unlike traditional dieting methods that prescribe strict rules and restrictions, intuitive eating encourages individuals to cultivate a more attuned and compassionate relationship with food and their bodies. Let's delve deeper into this concept:

1. **Understanding Intuitive Eating:**
   - Intuitive eating is an approach to eating that was developed by dietitians Evelyn Tribole and Elyse Resch. It is based on the premise that the body has innate wisdom and knows how to regulate food intake and maintain a healthy weight when given the opportunity to do so.
   - Intuitive eating involves rejecting the diet mentality and letting go of rigid food rules, restrictions, and judgments. Instead, it encourages individuals to tune into their body's natural hunger and fullness

cues, honor their cravings and preferences, and eat in a way that feels satisfying and nourishing.

- The core principles of intuitive eating include rejecting the diet mentality, honoring hunger and fullness, making peace with food, challenging the food police, discovering the satisfaction factor, coping with emotions without using food, respecting your body, and gentle nutrition.

2. **Listening to Your Body's Hunger Cues:**

- Hunger cues are the body's way of signaling that it needs nourishment and energy. Learning to recognize and honor these cues is essential for practicing intuitive eating. Hunger may manifest as physical sensations such as stomach growling, lightheadedness, irritability, or difficulty concentrating.

- Pay attention to your body's hunger signals throughout the day, and aim to eat when you start to feel moderately hungry rather than waiting until you are overly hungry. This can help prevent overeating and promote a more balanced and satisfying eating experience.
- Remember that hunger is a normal and natural part of being

human, and it's okay to eat when you're hungry. Trusting your body's signals and responding to them with nourishing foods is key to developing a healthy relationship with food.

3. **Honoring Your Body's Fullness Cues:**
    - Fullness cues, also known as satiety cues, are the body's signals that it has had enough food and is satisfied. Learning to recognize and honor these cues is essential for practicing intuitive eating and preventing overeating.
    - Pay attention to how your body feels as you eat, and pause periodically to check in with your

level of fullness. Aim to stop eating when you feel comfortably satisfied, but not overly full or stuffed.

- Practice mindful eating by savoring each bite, chewing slowly, and paying attention to the taste, texture, and aroma of your food. This can help you tune into your body's signals of fullness and prevent mindless overeating.

4. **Cultivating Mindful Eating Practices:**

- Mindful eating is a key component of intuitive eating and involves bringing awareness and attention to the present moment while eating. It encourages individuals to eat with intention, attention, and curiosity, without judgment or distraction.

- Practice mindful eating by turning off distractions such as television, smartphones, or reading material, and focusing solely on the sensory experience of eating. Notice the colors, textures, aromas, and flavors of your food, and savor each bite with gratitude and appreciation.
- Use mindfulness techniques such as deep breathing, body scans, or guided imagery to center yourself before meals and connect with your body's hunger and fullness cues.

In summary, exploring the concept of intuitive eating and listening to your body's hunger and fullness cues can help you develop a healthier and more sustainable approach to eating. By trusting your body's innate wisdom and honoring its signals of hunger and fullness, you can cultivate a more attuned and compassionate relationship with food and your body. Practicing mindful eating and self-awareness techniques can support this process and help you reconnect with the joy and pleasure of eating, free from guilt, shame, or judgment. Remember that intuitive eating is a journey, and it's okay to seek support and guidance along the way as you navigate this transformative approach to nourishment and well-being

CHAPTER 5
MAKING INFORMED FOOD CHOICES IN A BUSY WORLD

Navigating the Grocery Store Aisles With Confidence and Discernment

Navigating the grocery store aisles with confidence and discernment is essential for making informed choices that align with your nutritional goals, preferences, and budget. With the vast array of products available, it's important to approach grocery shopping with intention, mindfulness, and a basic understanding of nutrition. Here are some tips for navigating the grocery store aisles with confidence:

1. **Create a Shopping List:**
   - Before heading to the grocery store, take some time to plan your meals and snacks for the week and create a shopping list based on your meal plan. Having a list helps you stay focused and

organized while shopping and reduces the likelihood of impulse purchases.

2. **Shop the Perimeter:**
   - In many grocery stores, the perimeter is where you'll find fresh produce, lean proteins, dairy products, and whole grains. These are the foundation of a healthy diet, so start your shopping trip by exploring the perimeter aisles first.
   - Fill your cart with a variety of colorful fruits and vegetables, lean cuts of meat or fish, eggs, dairy or plant-based milk alternatives, and whole grain bread or pasta.

3. **Read Food Labels:**

- When choosing packaged foods, take the time to read food labels and ingredient lists to make informed choices. Pay attention to serving sizes, calorie counts, macronutrient breakdowns (fat, protein, carbohydrates), and ingredient quality.
- Look for products with minimal added sugars, unhealthy fats, and artificial additives. Choose whole foods whenever possible and opt for products with recognizable ingredients that you can pronounce.

4. **Focus on Whole Foods:**
- Aim to fill your cart with primarily whole, minimally processed foods

that are nutrient-dense and provide essential vitamins, minerals, fiber, and antioxidants. These include fruits, vegetables, whole grains, lean proteins, nuts, seeds, and legumes.
- Limit your intake of highly processed and packaged foods that are high in added sugars, unhealthy fats, sodium, and artificial ingredients. While some packaged foods can be convenient, it's important to prioritize whole foods as the foundation of your diet.

5. **Be Mindful of Portion Sizes:**
- Pay attention to portion sizes when selecting items such as

grains, meats, and snacks. While
these foods can be nutritious,
overconsumption can lead to
excess calorie intake and weight
gain.

○ Use visual cues and portion size
guidelines to help you estimate
appropriate serving sizes. For
example, a serving of meat or fish
is about the size of your palm, a
serving of grains is about the size
of your fist, and a serving of
cheese is about the size of your
thumb.

6. **Shop Seasonally and Locally:**
○ Take advantage of seasonal
produce by choosing fruits and
vegetables that are in season. Not

only are seasonal produce items fresher and more flavorful, but they're also often more affordable and support local farmers and producers.

- Consider visiting farmers' markets or joining a community-supported agriculture (CSA) program to access fresh, locally grown produce and support sustainable agriculture practices.

7. **Compare Prices and Quality:**
   - Compare prices and quality when selecting products to ensure you're getting the best value for your money. Consider factors such as price per unit or ounce, nutritional value, and ingredient

quality when making purchasing decisions.

- Keep in mind that higher prices don't always equate to better quality, so be discerning in your choices and prioritize products that offer the best combination of value and nutrition.

8. **Be Flexible and Adventurous:**

- While it's important to have a plan and stick to your shopping list, don't be afraid to be flexible and open to trying new foods or recipes. Explore different aisles and sections of the grocery store to discover new ingredients and flavors that can add variety and excitement to your meals.

○ Challenge yourself to incorporate a new fruit, vegetable, grain, or protein source into your shopping cart each week to expand your culinary repertoire and support a diverse and balanced diet.

By following these tips, you can navigate the grocery store aisles with confidence and discernment, making choices that support your health, well-being, and nutritional goals. With a little planning, mindfulness, and knowledge, you can shop with confidence and fill your cart with nourishing foods that nourish your body and delight your taste buds.

Decoding Food Labels and Marketing Claims to Make Informed Purchasing Decisions

Decoding food labels and marketing claims is essential for making informed purchasing decisions and selecting products that align with your nutritional goals, dietary preferences, and health needs. In today's food landscape, where packaging and marketing can often be misleading, it's important to understand how to navigate food labels and interpret the information provided. Let's explore the key components of food labels and marketing claims and how to decipher them effectively:

1. **Understanding the Basics of Food Labels:**
    - Food labels provide valuable information about the nutritional content of packaged foods, including serving sizes, calorie counts, macronutrient breakdowns (fat, protein, carbohydrates), and ingredient lists.
    - Pay attention to the serving size listed on the label, as all of the nutritional information is based on this serving size. Be mindful of portion sizes and adjust accordingly to avoid overconsumption.

o Familiarize yourself with the different sections of a food label, including the Nutrition Facts panel, ingredient list, and any additional claims or certifications displayed on the packaging.

2. **Interpreting the Nutrition Facts Panel:**

o The Nutrition Facts panel provides detailed information about the nutritional content of a food product, including the amount of calories, macronutrients, vitamins, minerals, and other nutrients per serving.

o Look for key nutrients such as fiber, vitamins, and minerals that contribute to overall health and well-being. Aim to choose foods that are rich in nutrients and low in added sugars, unhealthy fats, sodium, and artificial additives.

- Pay attention to the % Daily Value (% DV) listed on the Nutrition Facts panel, which indicates how much of a particular nutrient one serving of the food contributes to your daily recommended intake based on a 2,000-calorie diet. Use this as a guide to make informed choices about nutrient-rich foods.

3. **Reading the Ingredient List:**

- The ingredient list provides insight into the composition of a food product and the quality of its ingredients. Ingredients are listed in descending order by weight, with the most abundant ingredients listed first.

- Scan the ingredient list for whole, minimally processed ingredients and avoid products with long lists of artificial additives, preservatives, colors, and flavors. Choose products with recognizable ingredients that you can pronounce and understand.

4. **Deciphering Marketing Claims and Labels:**

- Be critical of marketing claims and labels that may be misleading or exaggerated. Terms such as "natural," "healthy," "low-fat," "organic," and "gluten-free" are often used to attract consumers, but their meaning can vary depending on regulatory standards and definitions.

o Look for third-party certifications and seals of approval from reputable organizations such as the USDA Organic seal, Non-GMO Project Verified seal, Certified Gluten-Free seal, and Heart-Check mark from the American Heart Association. These certifications indicate that the product has met specific criteria and standards set forth by independent organizations.

5. Being Skeptical of Health Claims:

- Be skeptical of health claims that promise quick fixes or miraculous results. Claims such as "fat-free," "sugar-free," "low-carb," and "diet" may not always equate to healthier options and can sometimes be misleading.
- Avoid products that make bold health claims without providing substantial evidence to support their claims. Look for products that focus on overall nutritional quality and provide balanced, wholesome ingredients.

6. Doing Your Own Research:

- Take the time to research unfamiliar ingredients, additives, and processing methods to better understand their impact on health and well-being. Use reputable sources such as scientific journals, nutrition websites, and government agencies to gather information and make informed decisions.
- Consider consulting with a registered dietitian or nutritionist for personalized guidance and recommendations tailored to your individual health goals and dietary needs.

In summary, decoding food labels and marketing claims is a critical skill for making informed purchasing decisions and selecting foods that support health and well-being. By understanding the basics of food labels, interpreting the Nutrition Facts panel and ingredient list, and being skeptical of marketing claims, you can navigate the grocery store aisles with confidence and discernment. Remember to prioritize whole, minimally processed foods, and choose products that align with your nutritional goals and values. With practice and knowledge, you can become a savvy consumer and make choices that promote a balanced and nourishing diet.

Offering Practical Strategies for Dining out, Traveling, and Managing Social Situations While Staying True to Your Health Goals

Offering practical strategies for dining out, traveling, and managing social situations while staying true to your health goals is essential for maintaining a balanced and sustainable approach to nutrition and well-being. While these situations can present challenges, with careful planning, mindfulness, and flexibility, it's possible to navigate them successfully while still enjoying delicious food and social experiences. Here are some practical strategies for each scenario:

1. **Dining Out:**

- Review the Menu in Advance: Before dining out, take a look at the menu online if available. Look for healthier options such as grilled or roasted proteins, salads, vegetable-based dishes, and whole grain options. Avoid dishes that are fried, breaded, or heavy in cream-based sauces.

- Modify Your Order: Don't be afraid to ask for modifications to suit your dietary preferences or restrictions. Request items to be grilled instead of fried, served with sauce on the side, or substituted with additional vegetables instead of starches.

- Practice Portion Control: Restaurant portions are often larger than necessary. Consider sharing an entree with a friend, ordering a smaller appetizer or starter as your main dish, or asking for a to-go box to portion out half of your meal before you start eating.
- Be Mindful of Extras: Be cautious of extras like bread baskets, appetizers, and desserts, as they can add extra calories and contribute to overeating. If you do indulge, try to balance it out with lighter choices during the main course.
- Stay Hydrated: Opt for water or unsweetened beverages instead of sugary drinks or alcoholic beverages,

which can add extra calories and contribute to dehydration. Limit alcohol consumption and alternate between alcoholic and non-alcoholic drinks.

2. **Traveling:**

- Pack Healthy Snacks: Bring along nutritious snacks such as nuts, seeds, fruit, whole grain crackers, or protein bars to have on hand while traveling. This can help you avoid unhealthy food choices at airports, gas stations, or convenience stores.
- Research Dining Options: Before traveling to a new destination, research local restaurants, markets, and grocery stores that offer healthy and nutritious options. Look for

restaurants that focus on fresh, locally sourced ingredients and offer a variety of dietary options.

- Stay Active: Incorporate physical activity into your travel plans by exploring the area on foot, renting bikes, or seeking out hiking trails or outdoor activities. Staying active can help offset any indulgences and keep you feeling energized during your trip.

- Practice Moderation: While it's okay to enjoy local cuisine and treats while traveling, try to practice moderation and balance your indulgences with healthier choices. Choose smaller portions, share meals with others, and focus on savoring the experience rather than overindulging.

3. **Managing Social Situations:**
- Communicate Your Needs: If you have specific dietary restrictions or preferences, communicate them to your friends, family, or hosts in advance. Offer to bring a dish that fits your dietary needs or suggest restaurants that offer options for everyone.
- Focus on Socializing: Instead of making food the primary focus of social gatherings, emphasize the social aspect of spending time with friends and loved ones. Engage in activities such as walking, hiking,

playing sports, or enjoying a picnic in the park.

- Plan Ahead: If you know you'll be attending a social event with limited healthy options, eat a balanced meal beforehand to help curb your appetite and prevent overeating. Bring along nutritious snacks or eat a small, healthy snack beforehand to avoid arriving overly hungry.
- Be Flexible: Remember that it's okay to deviate from your usual eating routine occasionally for special occasions or social events. Practice flexibility and forgiveness if you veer off track, and focus on making healthier choices when possible without feeling guilty.

By implementing these practical strategies for dining out, traveling, and managing social situations, you can stay true to your health goals while still enjoying delicious food and meaningful social experiences. Remember to prioritize balance, moderation, and mindfulness in your approach to eating, and don't forget to savor the moments and enjoy the company of those around you. With a little planning and flexibility, you can navigate these situations successfully and maintain a healthy and fulfilling lifestyle.

CHAPTER 6
CULTIVATING SUSTAINABLE LIFESTYLE HABIT

Recognizing the Interconnectedness of Nutrition, Physical Activity, Sleep, Stress Management, and Overall Well-being

Recognizing the interconnectedness of nutrition, physical activity, sleep, stress management, and overall well-being is fundamental to achieving optimal health and vitality. These aspects of wellness are deeply intertwined, with each one influencing and supporting the others in a complex and dynamic relationship. By understanding how these factors interact and impact one another, individuals can take a holistic approach to their health and well-being, leading to greater balance, resilience, and vitality. Let's explore the interconnectedness of these key components:

1. **Nutrition:**
   - Nutrition plays a foundational role in overall health and well-being, providing the body with essential nutrients for energy, growth, repair, and maintenance. A balanced and varied diet that includes a wide range of fruits, vegetables, whole grains, lean proteins, and healthy fats

supports optimal physical and mental function.
- Nutrient-rich foods provide the building blocks for cellular function, immune function, hormone regulation, and neurotransmitter production, influencing mood, energy levels, cognitive function, and overall vitality.

2. **Physical Activity:**
- Regular physical activity is essential for maintaining physical fitness, cardiovascular health, muscle strength, flexibility, and endurance. Exercise also supports mental well-being by reducing stress, anxiety, and

depression, improving mood, cognitive function, and self-esteem.

- Physical activity stimulates the release of endorphins, neurotransmitters, and growth factors that promote feelings of happiness, relaxation, and overall well-being. It also enhances circulation, oxygenation, and nutrient delivery to tissues, supporting overall vitality and longevity.

3. **Sleep**:

- Quality sleep is crucial for physical and mental health, providing the body with essential rest and recovery time. Adequate sleep supports immune function, hormone regulation, metabolism, cognitive function, and emotional resilience.

- Sleep deprivation can lead to a variety of health issues, including impaired cognitive function, mood disturbances, weakened immune function, weight gain, and increased risk of chronic diseases such as diabetes, heart disease, and depression.

4. **Stress Management:**

- Chronic stress can have profound effects on health and well-being, contributing to inflammation, immune dysfunction, hormonal imbalances, and increased risk of chronic diseases. Effective stress management techniques such as mindfulness, meditation, deep breathing, yoga, and relaxation techniques can help mitigate the negative effects of stress on the body and mind.

- Stress reduction promotes a state of relaxation and calmness, supporting optimal physiological function, immune response, and overall well-being. It also enhances resilience to stressors, allowing individuals to cope more effectively with life's challenges.

5. **Overall Well-being:**

- The interconnectedness of nutrition, physical activity, sleep, and stress management contributes to overall well-being and vitality. When these factors are in balance, individuals experience greater energy, vitality, resilience, and overall quality of life.

- Taking a holistic approach to health involves prioritizing self-care practices that support physical, mental, and emotional well-being. This includes nourishing the body with nutritious foods, engaging in regular physical activity, prioritizing restful sleep, practicing stress management techniques, and fostering positive social connections and relationships.

By recognizing the interconnectedness of nutrition, physical activity, sleep, stress management, and overall well-being, individuals can take a holistic approach to their health that addresses the underlying factors contributing to wellness. By prioritizing self-care practices that support optimal functioning of the body and mind, individuals can enhance their quality of life, resilience, and vitality for years to come.

Providing Evidence-based Recommendations for Incorporating Movement, Relaxation techniques, and Self-care Practices into your Daily Routine

Incorporating movement, relaxation techniques, and self-care practices into your daily routine is essential for promoting physical, mental, and emotional well-being. These practices help reduce stress, improve mood, enhance resilience, and support overall health and vitality. By prioritizing self-care activities that nurture your body, mind, and spirit, you can cultivate a greater sense of balance, fulfillment, and resilience in your daily life. Let's explore evidence-based recommendations for incorporating movement, relaxation techniques, and self-care practices into your daily routine:

1. **Movement:**
   - Aim for Regular Physical Activity: Engage in moderate-intensity aerobic activity for at least 150 minutes per week, or vigorous-intensity aerobic activity for at least 75 minutes per week, according to the recommendations from the Centers for Disease Control and Prevention (CDC). This can include activities such as brisk walking, jogging,

swimming, cycling, dancing, or participating in group fitness classes.

- Incorporate Strength Training: Include strength training exercises at least two days per week to target major muscle groups. Strength training helps improve muscle strength, endurance, and bone density, while also supporting metabolism and overall physical function.
- Find Activities You Enjoy: Choose activities that you enjoy and that fit your interests, preferences, and lifestyle. Whether it's hiking in nature, practicing yoga, playing sports, or dancing to your favorite music, find

ways to make movement enjoyable and sustainable.

2. **Relaxation Techniques:**

- Practice Mindfulness Meditation: Dedicate time each day to mindfulness meditation, focusing on the present moment with acceptance and without judgment. Mindfulness meditation has been shown to reduce stress, anxiety, and depression, while also improving attention, emotional regulation, and overall well-being.

- Deep Breathing Exercises: Incorporate deep breathing exercises into your daily routine to promote relaxation and stress relief. Practice diaphragmatic breathing, belly breathing, or progressive muscle relaxation to activate the body's relaxation response and reduce physiological arousal.

- Progressive Muscle Relaxation (PMR): Practice PMR by systematically tensing and relaxing different muscle groups in the body, starting from the feet and working your way up to the head. PMR helps release tension, reduce muscle stiffness, and promote physical and mental relaxation.

3. **Self-Care Practices:**

- Prioritize Sleep: Make sleep a priority by aiming for 7-9 hours of quality sleep per night. Create a relaxing bedtime routine, establish a consistent sleep schedule, and create a sleep-friendly environment that promotes restful sleep.

- Nourish Your Body: Eat a balanced and nutritious diet that provides essential nutrients for optimal health and well-being. Include a variety of fruits, vegetables, whole grains, lean proteins, and healthy fats in your meals, and stay hydrated by drinking plenty of water throughout the day.
- Set Boundaries: Learn to say no to activities or commitments that drain your energy or cause unnecessary stress. Set boundaries to protect your time, energy, and well-being, and prioritize activities that align with your values, priorities, and goals.

4. **Integration into Daily Routine:**

- Schedule Time for Self-Care: Set aside dedicated time each day for self-care activities, whether it's in the morning, during lunch breaks, or in the evening before bed. Treat self-care as a non-negotiable part of your daily routine, just like brushing your teeth or eating meals.
- Combine Activities: Look for opportunities to combine movement, relaxation techniques, and self-care practices throughout your day. For example, you could go for a walk in nature while practicing mindfulness, or practice deep breathing exercises during your daily commute or before bedtime.

- Be Flexible: Be flexible and adaptable in your approach to self-care, recognizing that life can be unpredictable and that priorities may shift from day to day. Be kind to yourself and adjust your self-care practices as needed to accommodate changing circumstances and demands.

By incorporating evidence-based recommendations for movement, relaxation techniques, and self-care practices into your daily routine, you can nurture your physical, mental, and emotional well-being and cultivate a greater sense of balance, resilience, and vitality in your life. Remember that self-care is not selfish, but rather an essential aspect of maintaining health and happiness for yourself and those around you. Prioritize your well-being and make time for self-care activities that nourish your body, mind, and spirit each day.

Empowering you to Make Sustainable Lifestyle Changes that Support your Health and Vitality for the Long Haul

Empowering yourself to make sustainable lifestyle changes that support your health and vitality for the long haul is a transformative journey that requires commitment, self-awareness, and a willingness to prioritize your well-being. Sustainable lifestyle changes involve adopting habits and behaviors that promote overall health, resilience, and vitality while considering long-term implications and outcomes. By taking a holistic approach to health and well-being and implementing evidence-based strategies, you can create lasting change that enhances your quality of life and supports your long-term health goals. Here's an extensive guide on how to empower yourself to make sustainable lifestyle changes:

1. **Define Your Health Goals:**
   - Take some time to reflect on your current health status, values, priorities, and aspirations. Identify specific health goals that are meaningful to you and align with your values and aspirations.
   - Break down your goals into smaller, actionable steps that are realistic, achievable, and measurable. Set clear timelines and benchmarks to

track your progress and celebrate your successes along the way.

2. **Cultivate Self-Awareness:**
   - Develop self-awareness by tuning into your thoughts, emotions, behaviors, and habits related to health and well-being. Pay attention to your body's signals, needs, and responses to different lifestyle factors.
   - Reflect on your motivations, triggers, barriers, and patterns of behavior related to nutrition, physical activity, sleep, stress management, and self-care. Identify areas where you can make positive changes and commit to taking proactive steps towards improvement.

3. **Educate Yourself:**
  - Seek out reliable sources of information and evidence-based resources to learn more about nutrition, exercise, sleep, stress management, and other aspects of health and well-being. Stay informed about current research, trends, and best practices in health promotion and disease prevention.
  - Take advantage of reputable websites, books, podcasts, courses, and educational programs that provide practical tips, strategies, and insights for improving your health and vitality.

4. **Set Realistic Expectations:**

- Recognize that sustainable lifestyle changes take time, effort, and persistence to achieve. Be patient with yourself and set realistic expectations for progress and outcomes.
- Focus on making gradual, sustainable changes that are manageable and maintainable over the long term, rather than seeking quick fixes or drastic measures that may not be sustainable or healthy.

5. **Develop Healthy Habits:**

- Focus on building healthy habits that support your health and well-being on a daily basis. Incorporate habits such as eating a balanced diet, engaging in regular physical activity,

prioritizing sleep, managing stress
effectively, and practicing self-care
rituals.

- Start small and gradually increase
the complexity or intensity of your
habits over time. Consistency is key
to establishing new habits, so aim to
practice them regularly and
incorporate them into your daily
routine.

6. **Cultivate Resilience:**

- Develop resilience by adopting a
growth mindset and viewing
challenges and setbacks as
opportunities for learning and growth.
Embrace setbacks as natural parts of
the process and use them as

opportunities to reassess and adjust your approach.

- Build coping skills and strategies for managing stress, adversity, and setbacks effectively. Practice self-compassion, optimism, gratitude, and mindfulness to cultivate resilience and bounce back from challenges with greater strength and resilience.

7. **Build a Support System:**

- Surround yourself with supportive individuals who encourage and empower you to prioritize your health and well-being. Share your goals, challenges, and successes with friends, family members, or peers who can provide encouragement, accountability, and practical support.

- Seek out professional support from healthcare providers, therapists, nutritionists, personal trainers, or health coaches who can offer guidance, expertise, and personalized recommendations to help you achieve your health goals.

8. **Monitor Your Progress:**
   - Track your progress regularly by monitoring your behaviors, habits, and outcomes related to health and well-being. Keep a journal, use a mobile app, or create a spreadsheet to record your daily activities, progress, and achievements.
   - Evaluate your progress periodically and adjust your approach as needed based on your results and feedback.

Celebrate your successes, no matter how small, and use them as motivation to continue moving forward towards your goals.

9. **Practice Self-Compassion:**
   - Be kind to yourself and practice self-compassion as you navigate the ups and downs of making lifestyle changes. Acknowledge your efforts, progress, and achievements, and be gentle with yourself during times of struggle or setbacks.
   - Let go of perfectionism and unrealistic expectations, and embrace the journey of self-improvement with patience, acceptance, and self-love.

10. **Embrace Long-Term Perspective:**

- Adopt a long-term perspective on health and well-being, recognizing that sustainable lifestyle changes are a lifelong journey rather than a quick fix. Focus on creating habits and behaviors that support your health and vitality for the long haul.
- Stay committed to your health goals and prioritize self-care as an ongoing practice that evolves and adapts with you over time. Remember that every positive choice you make contributes to your overall well-being and sets the foundation for a healthier, happier future.

By following these evidence-based recommendations and empowering yourself to make sustainable lifestyle changes, you can enhance your health, vitality, and quality of life for the long term. Embrace the journey of self-discovery, growth, and transformation, and commit to prioritizing your health and well-being as a lifelong investment in yourself. With dedication, perseverance, and self-compassion, you can create a life that is vibrant, fulfilling, and deeply nourishing on all levels.

CHAPTER 7
OVERCOMING CHALLENGES AND STAYING MOTIVATED

Identifying Common Obstacles to Healthy Eating and Weight Management

Identifying common obstacles to healthy eating and weight management is crucial for overcoming challenges and achieving long-term success in maintaining a balanced diet and healthy weight. While everyone's journey is unique, there are several common obstacles that individuals may encounter along the way. By recognizing these obstacles and understanding how they can impact eating behaviors and weight management efforts, individuals can develop effective strategies to address them and cultivate healthier habits. Let's delve into these obstacles in detail:

1. **Unhealthy Eating Habits:**
   - Emotional Eating: Many individuals turn to food for comfort, stress relief, or distraction from negative emotions. Emotional eating can lead to overeating and weight gain, as food becomes a coping mechanism for dealing with difficult emotions.
   - Mindless Eating: Eating while distracted, such as watching TV, working, or scrolling through your

phone, can lead to overconsumption and a lack of awareness of hunger and fullness cues.

- Poor Food Choices: A diet high in processed foods, sugary snacks, and unhealthy fats can contribute to weight gain, poor nutritional status, and increased risk of chronic diseases.

2. **Environmental Factors:**

- Food Availability: Easy access to unhealthy foods, such as fast food, vending machines, and convenience stores, can make it challenging to make healthy choices, especially when faced with time constraints or limited options.

- Food Marketing: The pervasive marketing of unhealthy foods, especially to children and adolescents, can influence food preferences, cravings, and consumption habits, making it difficult to resist tempting but unhealthy options.
- Social Pressures: Social gatherings, parties, and celebrations often revolve around food and can present challenges in making healthy choices, especially when faced with peer pressure or social norms that encourage overindulgence.

3. **Psychological Factors:**
- Perfectionism: Striving for perfection in eating habits or body image can

lead to rigid dieting behaviors, self-criticism, and feelings of failure when unable to meet unrealistic expectations.

- Negative Self-Talk: Negative thoughts and beliefs about oneself, body image, and eating habits can undermine self-esteem, motivation, and confidence in making healthy choices.
- Lack of Self-Efficacy: Doubts about one's ability to make lasting changes or overcome obstacles can lead to feelings of helplessness, resignation, and avoidance of healthy behaviors.

4. **Lifestyle Challenges:**
- Time Constraints: Busy schedules, work commitments, and family

responsibilities can make it challenging to prioritize meal planning, grocery shopping, and cooking nutritious meals at home.

- Financial Constraints: Limited budget or financial resources may restrict access to fresh, healthy foods and make it difficult to afford nutritious options, especially in low-income communities.
- Lack of Social Support: Limited support from family, friends, or community members can hinder efforts to make healthy changes, as social support plays a crucial role in motivation, accountability, and behavior change.

5. **Physiological Factors:**

- Metabolic Factors: Individual differences in metabolism, hormones, and genetic predispositions can influence weight management efforts, making it easier or harder for some individuals to lose or maintain weight.
- Gut Health: Imbalances in gut microbiota and digestive health can affect appetite regulation, nutrient absorption, and metabolism, potentially contributing to weight gain or difficulty in losing weight.
- Sleep Disturbances: Inadequate sleep or poor sleep quality can disrupt hormone regulation, appetite control, and energy balance, leading

to increased hunger, cravings, and
weight gain over time.

6. **Unrealistic Expectations:**
   - Fad Diets: The allure of quick-fix
     diets and weight loss programs
     promising rapid results can lead to
     unrealistic expectations,
     disappointment, and frustration when
     unsustainable or unsustainable
     methods fail to deliver long-term
     success.
   - Comparing to Others: Comparing
     oneself to others or unrealistic
     standards portrayed in media can
     create feelings of inadequacy,
     insecurity, and dissatisfaction with
     one's body or progress, undermining

confidence and motivation to make healthy changes.

By identifying these common obstacles to healthy eating and weight management, individuals can develop personalized strategies to overcome challenges and foster sustainable habits that support their long-term health and well-being. These strategies may include seeking professional support from a registered dietitian, therapist, or health coach, practicing mindfulness and self-compassion, creating a supportive environment that promotes healthy choices, and focusing on small, achievable goals that align with personal values and priorities. With dedication, perseverance, and support, individuals can overcome obstacles and achieve lasting success in maintaining a balanced diet and healthy weight for life.

Offering Practical Solutions for Overcoming Setbacks, Managing Cravings, and Staying Motivated on your Journey

Offering practical solutions for overcoming setbacks, managing cravings, and staying motivated on your health and wellness journey is essential for maintaining momentum and achieving long-term success. Setbacks are a natural part of the process, and managing cravings and staying motivated can be challenging at times. However, with the right strategies and mindset, individuals can navigate these obstacles effectively and stay on track towards their goals. Here are practical solutions for overcoming setbacks, managing cravings, and staying motivated:

1. **Overcoming Setbacks:**
   - Practice Resilience: View setbacks as opportunities for learning and growth rather than reasons to give up. Cultivate resilience by reframing setbacks as temporary obstacles and focusing on finding solutions and lessons learned.
   - Identify Triggers: Reflect on the factors that contributed to the setback, such as stress, emotional triggers, or environmental cues. Identify patterns and triggers that may lead to unhealthy behaviors and

develop strategies to address them proactively.

- **Reassess Your Goals:** Reassess your goals and expectations to ensure they are realistic, achievable, and aligned with your values and priorities. Adjust your goals if necessary and break them down into smaller, manageable steps to prevent feeling overwhelmed.

2. **Managing Cravings:**

- **Mindful Eating:** Practice mindful eating by paying attention to hunger and fullness cues, as well as the taste, texture, and enjoyment of food. Slow down and savor each bite, and be mindful of emotional and environmental triggers that may trigger cravings.

- Stay Hydrated: Drink plenty of water throughout the day to stay hydrated and prevent dehydration, which can sometimes be mistaken for hunger. Opt for water or unsweetened beverages instead of sugary drinks or caffeinated beverages that can exacerbate cravings.

- Choose Healthy Alternatives: When cravings strike, opt for healthier alternatives that satisfy your cravings while still aligning with your health goals. For example, choose a piece of fruit, a handful of nuts, or a small serving of dark chocolate instead of sugary snacks or processed foods.

3. **Staying Motivated:**
- Set Meaningful Goals: Set goals that are meaningful, inspiring, and aligned with your values and aspirations. Focus on intrinsic motivations, such as improved health, increased energy, or enhanced quality of life, rather than external rewards or outcomes.
- Celebrate Progress: Celebrate your progress and achievements, no matter how small. Recognize and acknowledge your efforts and successes along the way, and use them as motivation to keep moving forward towards your goals.
- Find Support: Surround yourself with supportive individuals who

encourage and empower you to prioritize your health and well-being. Share your goals, challenges, and successes with friends, family members, or peers who can provide encouragement, accountability, and practical support.

4. **Practice Self-Compassion:**
- Be Kind to Yourself: Practice self-compassion and kindness towards yourself, especially during times of setbacks or challenges. Treat yourself with the same compassion and understanding that you would offer to a friend, and avoid self-criticism or negative self-talk.
- Forgive Yourself: Let go of perfectionism and forgive yourself for

mistakes or slip-ups along the way. Recognize that setbacks are a natural part of the process and an opportunity for growth and learning, rather than a reflection of your worth or ability.

5. **Stay Consistent:**

- Create a Routine: Establish a regular routine that includes healthy eating, physical activity, sleep, and self-care practices. Stick to your routine as much as possible, even during times of stress or disruption, to maintain consistency and momentum towards your goals.

- Focus on Progress, Not Perfection: Shift your focus from perfection to progress, recognizing that small, consistent changes over time can lead to significant improvements in health and well-being. Celebrate each step forward and use setbacks as opportunities to learn and grow.

By implementing these practical solutions for overcoming setbacks, managing cravings, and staying motivated, individuals can navigate the ups and downs of their health and wellness journey with resilience, determination, and self-compassion. Remember that setbacks are temporary, cravings are manageable, and motivation can be cultivated through meaningful goals, support, and self-care practices. With dedication, perseverance, and a positive mindset, individuals can overcome obstacles and achieve lasting success in prioritizing their health and well-being.

Fostering a Supportive Community and Mindset of Self-compassion, Resilience, and Perseverance

Fostering a supportive community and mindset of self-compassion, resilience, and perseverance is essential for creating a nurturing environment that empowers individuals to thrive and overcome challenges on their journey towards health and well-being. Building connections with others who share similar goals, values, and experiences can provide encouragement, accountability, and inspiration, while cultivating self-compassion, resilience, and perseverance enables individuals to navigate setbacks and adversity with strength and grace. Here's how to foster a supportive community and mindset of self-compassion, resilience, and perseverance:

1. **Cultivate a Supportive Community:**
   - Build Connections: Seek out like-minded individuals who share similar goals and values related to health and well-being. Join support groups, online communities, or local meet-ups focused on nutrition, fitness, mindfulness, or personal development.
   - Share Your Journey: Open up and share your journey, challenges, and successes with others in your community. Be authentic and

vulnerable, and offer support and encouragement to others who may be facing similar struggles or obstacles.

- Seek Accountability: Find an accountability partner or group to help you stay on track towards your goals. Check in regularly, set goals together, and celebrate each other's progress and achievements along the way.

2. Cultivate a Mindset of Self-Compassion:

- Practice Self-Kindness: Treat yourself with kindness, understanding, and acceptance, especially during times of difficulty or setback. Offer yourself the same compassion and support that you would offer to a friend in need.

- Embrace Imperfection: Let go of perfectionism and embrace the imperfections and challenges that are a natural part of the human experience. Recognize that it's okay to make mistakes, experience setbacks, and fall short of your expectations at times.
- Practice Mindfulness: Cultivate mindfulness by staying present in the moment and observing your thoughts and feelings without judgment. Notice any self-critical or negative thoughts that arise and gently redirect them with self-compassion and kindness.

3. **Cultivate Resilience:**
- Adapt to Change: Embrace change as an opportunity for growth and adaptation, rather than a threat to your well-being. Develop flexibility and adaptability in the face of adversity, and focus on finding solutions and opportunities for learning and growth.
- Develop Coping Skills: Build a toolkit of coping skills and strategies for managing stress, adversity, and setbacks effectively. Practice relaxation techniques, mindfulness meditation, deep breathing, or progressive muscle relaxation to help calm your mind and body during times of stress.

- Find Meaning: Find meaning and purpose in your journey towards health and well-being. Connect with your values, passions, and aspirations, and let them guide you through challenges and difficult times with resilience and determination.

4. **Cultivate Perseverance:**

- Stay Committed: Stay committed to your goals and priorities, even when faced with obstacles, setbacks, or challenges. Remember why you started your journey in the first place and keep your vision and aspirations in mind as you persevere through difficulties.

- Focus on Progress: Focus on progress, not perfection, and

celebrate each step forward towards your goals. Break down your goals into smaller, manageable steps, and celebrate your achievements along the way.

- Stay Positive: Cultivate a positive mindset and outlook, even during difficult times. Practice gratitude, optimism, and self-belief, and surround yourself with positive influences and supportive people who uplift and inspire you.

By fostering a supportive community and mindset of self-compassion, resilience, and perseverance, individuals can navigate the challenges and obstacles on their journey towards health and well-being with greater strength, courage, and grace. Remember that you are not alone in your journey, and that together, we can support and uplift each other as we strive to create lives that are vibrant, fulfilling, and deeply nourishing on all levels.

In conclusion, our journey through Chapters 1 to 7 has been a profound exploration of the principles, strategies, and practices for nurturing holistic health and well-being. From understanding emotions and cultivating self-awareness to embracing nutrition, physical activity, stress management, and self-care, each chapter has offered valuable insights and practical tools for fostering a balanced and fulfilling life.

Chapter 1 laid the foundation by emphasizing the importance of understanding emotions and recognizing their influence on our behaviors, choices, and overall well-being. By cultivating self-awareness and emotional intelligence, we empower ourselves to make conscious decisions that support our health and vitality. Building upon this foundation, Chapters 2 and 3 delved into the intricacies of nutrition and physical activity, highlighting the importance of nourishing our bodies with wholesome foods and engaging in regular movement that promotes strength, flexibility, and vitality. By adopting a mindful and balanced approach to eating and exercise, we can optimize our health and energy levels while cultivating a positive relationship with our bodies.

In Chapters 4 and 5, we explored the significance of stress management and self-care in maintaining overall well-being. By prioritizing self-care practices such as mindfulness, relaxation techniques, and healthy lifestyle habits, we can enhance our resilience, reduce stress, and foster a greater sense of inner peace and balance.

Chapter 6 delved into the intricacies of sleep and its profound impact on our physical, mental, and emotional health. By prioritizing restorative sleep and adopting healthy sleep habits, we can optimize our cognitive function, mood regulation, and overall vitality.

Finally, in Chapter 7, we discussed the importance of cultivating a supportive community and mindset of self-compassion, resilience, and perseverance. By building connections with others who share our values and aspirations, we create a nurturing environment that empowers us to overcome challenges, celebrate successes, and thrive on our journey towards holistic health and well-being. As we conclude our exploration, let us carry forward the insights, wisdom, and practices gleaned from each chapter, knowing that our journey towards vibrant health and fulfillment is an ongoing process of growth and discovery. May we continue to prioritize self-care, nourish our bodies and minds with love and compassion, and support one another on this transformative journey towards a life that is vibrant, resilient, and deeply fulfilling in every way.

With gratitude and determination, let us embrace the path ahead with open hearts and steadfast commitment to our well-being, knowing that each step we take brings us closer to the vibrant, flourishing life we aspire to create.

This comprehensive conclusion encapsulates the key themes and takeaways from each chapter, providing a holistic overview of the journey towards holistic health and well-being.

9 799888 832665